Fertility Diet Manual for Beginners:

Full Guide on Fertility Diet to Boost Conception; Dos & Don'ts of Fertility Diet & the Common Mistakes to Avoid While Trying to Get Pregnant & So Much More

By

Dr. Bradley L. Jackson

Copyright@2020

TABLE OF CONTENTS

THE END

CHAPTER ONE

INTODUCTION

Fertility Diet

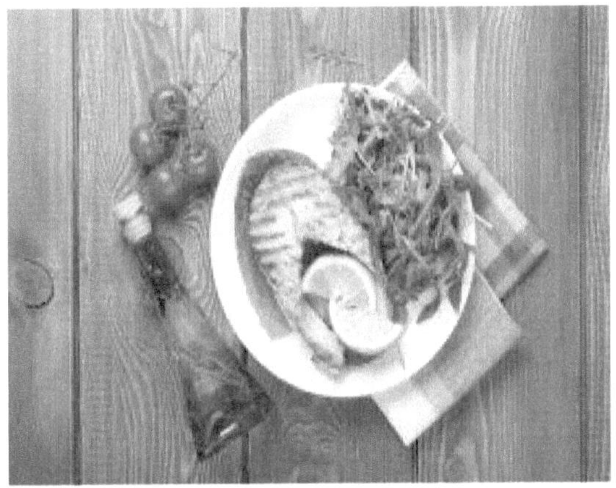

Fertility diet plan is a supportive component of preconception care. Understanding the impact certain foods have on fertility will aid to generate a plan that will improve your chances of natural conception

and a healthy pregnancy.

CHAPTER TWO

Fertility Diet Tips

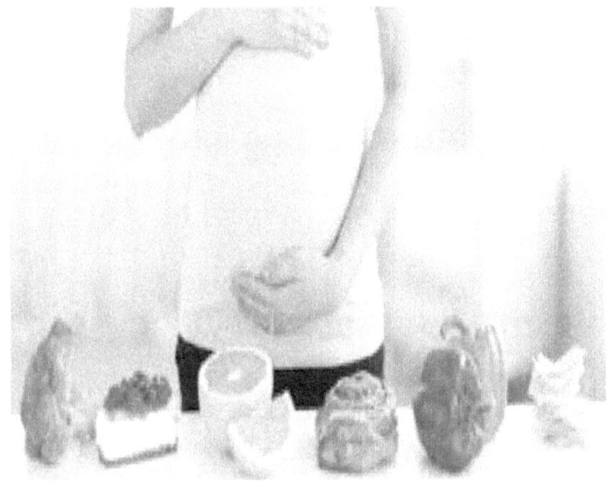

Stay away from sugary food and drink, such as biscuits, cake, sweet and fizzy drinks.

Make sure you eat five portions of different fruits and vegetables each day.

Don't skip breakfast, choosing cereal that contains no sugar.

Consume more unsaturated 'good' fats such as nuts avocado and seeds.

Sidestep saturated 'bad' fats, such as fried food, pies pastry and biscuits.

Note, make sure you avoid too much ready-prepared food too. The flavorings chemical preservatives and colorings that are added can affect the nutrients in the food.

CHAPTER THREE

Foods to Boost Your Odds of Conception and Quantity to Consume

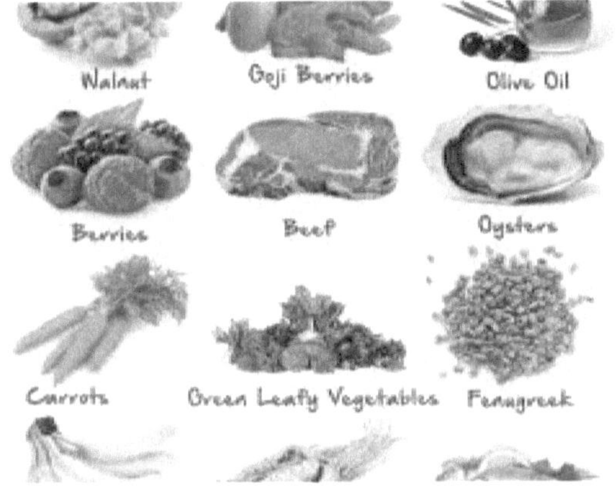

Consuming nutrient-rich diets is usually safer than concentrated supplements. The exception to this is with folic acid –most doctors recommend the intake of folic acid supplement when to get pregnant.

You can also have too much of a good thing. Except your doctor prescribes the intake of folic acid, your daily supplements intake shouldn't include more than 1,000 mcg folic acid.

Too much doses of folic acid may cover up a vitamin B-12 deficiency, and when not detected early can cause irreversible damage. Your B-12 levels should be tested by your doctor before putting you on high dose of folic acid supplement.

Many fertility super foods contain nutrients that are essential to fertility health. That is a good reason for us to add them to our diet.

So why are you still waiting? Let's check out the foods to boost our fertility.

> **Consume More Cow Liver for a Fertility Boost**

Liver gotten from cow is loaded with fertility-boosting nutrients.

Why Cow Liver May Increase Fertility

Cow liver contains many nutrients that are essential to the reproductive health.

One portion of cow liver contains (68 grams):

- Daily value of vitamin A is 431%
- Daily value of riboflavin is 137%
- Daily value of selenium is 35%
- Daily value of m 24% of zinc, a mineral that is essential for semen healthy
- It is naturally high in coenzyme Q10, which helps to boost egg quality and motility of semen

➢ **Boiled Tomatoes for Fertility**

Cooked tomatoes help to enhance your fertility.

Why Boiled Tomatoes May Increases Fertility

- Boiled tomatoes are rich in the nutrient lycopene, a great antioxidant.

- Lycopene is a powerful antioxidant, may increase sperm quantity, a study has suggested.

- It has been soon that supplementation of 4 to 8 mg of lycopene per day for 7to 12 months led to enhanced semen

health and increased the rate
of pregnancy.

How to consume it

Both boiled and raw tomatoes
contain lycopene, a cup of boiled
tomatoes is twice as much lycopene
as one cup of raw tomatoes.

You can opt for the boiled tomatoes
recipes. Tomatoes of any form are
still good for you!

➢ **Lentils and Beans for Fertility**

The consumption of lentils and beans
may help fertility. (All types of beans

go for boosting fertility but most especially black beans.)

High levels of polyamine and spermidine are found in lentils, they assistance sperm to fertilize the egg. They are also good source of folate. Folate which is also known as folic acid is an essential nutrient for conception and healthy embryos.

Lentils and beans are rich in fiber. Receiving enough fiber in your diet is a key to boost your hormone.

How to consume Lentils and Beans

One or two of your meat meals should be replaced with beans- based or lentil meals. You can as well throw some beans into your salad instead of meat or cheese.

> **Consume Asparagus for Fertility**

Boiled asparagus comprises tons of important nutrients.

Why Asparagus may Increase Fertility

Asparagus contains less calories but rich in vital nutrients to boost fertility.

A single cup of cooked asparagus will give you:

More than 60% of your daily value of folate

More than 20% of other vital nutrients like vitamin A, vitamin C, and vitamin thiamin.

Contains full daily value of vitamin K

Asparagus contains 8% of your daily zinc and 16% of your daily recommended amount of selenium, both are essential to boost male fertility

How to Consume Asparagus

Stay away from canned asparagus that contains lot of salt. If you choose to go for canned asparagus, go for low sodium options.

> ## Oysters for Fertility

Oysters, called an aphrodisiac, may also aid to boost fertility.

Why it May Increase Fertility

These fertility boosters appear on just about every fertility diet list. They are filled with fertility-boosting nutrients!

6 raw serving size of oysters contains only 139 calories, but rich in these essential reproductive minerals and vitamins:

Daily iron of 43%

Daily recommended value of vitamin B – 12 is 408%

Daily recommended value of selenium is 187%

Daily zinc of188%

How to Consume Oysters

Don't feel intimidated by the preparation of oysters. This dish can be easily prepared and served at home.

The healthiest option of consuming oysters is raw, but not everybody can do with raw oysters.

➢ **Walnuts**

Vital nutrients the body needs are found in walnuts.

Why it May Increase Fertility

Healthy fats are essential for healthy reproductive but also for overall health.   They are filled in omega – 3s and omega – 6s. It is the reason that led researchers to consider whether they might increase fertility. In a small but interesting study carried out, 117 men were unevenly allocated to 1 of 2 groups.

The control group, the men were told not to eat all tree nuts but continue their normal diet. While the experimental group, the men eat a premeasured packed of walnuts every day but also continue their normal diet.

Each package of walnut contained 75 grams ..The nut – eating group of men experienced improvements in semen health. Particularly, sperm vitality, Motility and morphology were improved.

How to Consume Walnuts

Make sure you replace your afternoon snack with a serving of walnuts.

➤ Egg as Fertility Booster

The yolk of egg benefits conception.

Why Yolk Increase Fertility

They are good source of B – vitamins. Which are vital for fertility, they are not cheap but are well worth it if you don't consume much fish.

They are also good source of lean protein, which has also been found to be good in boosting the fertility in male and female.

How to Consume Egg

Some nutrition specialists recommend eating just the whites of the egg and throwing out the yolk. Consume all of it. When you are trying to increase fertility, you need the nutrients present in the yolk.

When trying to lose weight, target cut back on calories elsewhere.

> ## Full – Fat Yogurt and Ice Cream to Increase Fertility

Prime your body for ovulation, by consuming lot of full – fat dairy products, like whole milk, ice cream, full – fat yogurt, cream cheese, and other cheese.

Why it May Increase Fertility

A study that was carried out found that women who consumed full – fat dairy products were less likely to experience problems from ovulation than women who consumed primarily low – fat dairy products.

How to Consume It

The best way to consume it is to switch to whole milk instead to of low – fat milk. (It becomes easy if you already have milk in your morning cereal or tea.)

Or, if you like taking yogurt, shift to – full fat yogurt in its place of the low – fat varieties.

Note, being overweight can affect fertility negatively, so don't take too much of it.

> **Consume Mature Cheeses to Increase Fertility**

Mature cheeses, like mature parmesan, cheddar, and manchego, may increase sperm fertility.

Why Cheese May Boost Fertility

Mature cheese contains polyamines. Pollyamines are essential proteins found in animal and plant products. They also occur naturally in human beings.

Research has proven that polyamines play an essential part in the reproductive system. Mature cheese is high in polyamine putrescine, which plays an important role in sperm health. It is also suspected that putrescine improves egg health, especially in women over 35 years of age.

How to Consume It

Be careful of the portion you add to your diet! Little amount of cheese contains lot of calories and saturated fat.

CHAPTER FOUR

Foods TO Avoid When Trying To Conceive

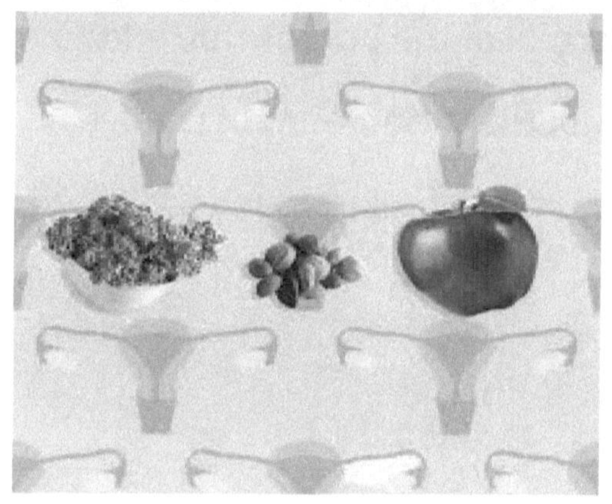

Consuming the right diet isn't always easy – especially when you are pregnant and looking at a whole new set of nutrition guidelines. Nevertheless even if you are just starting to think about conceiving, it is in right order to change some dietary.

Here are some critical foods you should stay away from when trying to get pregnant.

Don't be freak out if you have consumed any of these foods recently – their harm is in moderation. But to be safe, you have to keep these foods to a minimum when you are trying to get pregnant, and make sure you take them off your list once your test comes out positive.

Excess intake of Alcohol

CDC has recommended that women who could get pregnant to stay away from alcohol completely, but if you are to drink, Tolbert advises capping it at seven drinks each week. Alcohol contributes to infertility, and it reduces your body of vitamin B, which improves the odds of pregnancy and supports a fetus development.

Consuming Raw Animal Products

Seafood, egg, and raw meat might contain coliform salmonella which can infect a fetus if it gets entrance into the placenta. Ensure all animal products are well cooked.

Deli Meat

Processed meat like lunch meat and hot dogs, and also smoked fish, are susceptible to listeria contamination. If you want to consume deli meat, Fisher recommends heating it up until it's steaming to exterminate bacteria.

Consuming High – Mercury Fish

The human nervous system can be damaged by mercury, it means consuming mercury – rich seafood like tuna and swordfish while pregnant could harm your fetus directly. Consuming high – mercury fish before you getting pregnant could build up stores of mercury in your system, which could also affect the growth of the infant's nervous system. "Your baby's fetal nervous system is being formed before you even know you are pregnant." And it also reduces fertility rate.

Intake of Soda

Soda may also decrease fertility. " We think it's a mixture of the inflammation and metabolic changes which is caused by excess blood – sugar – spiking sweeteners and gut – bacteria – changing artificial sweeteners," Says Tolbert. Most soft drinks come in containers that have

BPA and other chemicals you might want to sidestep.

Trans Fats

Trans fats, can be seen in foods like microwave popcorns, baked goods prepared with shortening, and fried foods, can cause inflammation and resistance, which decrease fertility. Your blood vessels can be damaged, distracting the free flow of nutrients to the reproductive organ. Men should take it low on trans fats while they are trying to conceive because they reduce male sperm count and it's quantity.

Foods high – Glycemic – Index Foods

If you want to boost your fertility, step side foods that make your blood sugar spike, especially if you don't pair them with foods that decrease the rise. " Increase in blood sugar can cause inflammation, change our hormones, and impede ovulation," Choose slow burning

carbs, like whole – wheat bread and pasta or brown rice, over refined ones, make sure you combine them with protein, fiber, and healthy fats.

CHAPTER FIVE

Dos and Don'ts of fertility

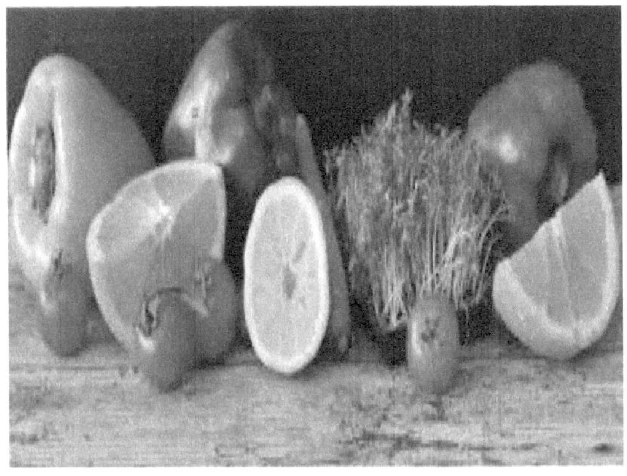

Your emotions run high when you are trying to conceive, and you feel confused when you start to think about what's next. The things to avoid and follow are:

Dos

Try to Seek Support

Infertility can be stressful; research has proven that the levels of stress in women that are infertile are equivalent to those women with AIDS, cancer or heart infection. The stress will not increase your chances of getting pregnant. Most women are not getting pregnant either, so a support group can help you. You can as well find an online infertility support groups, or ask your fertility specialist or doctor to recommend a local in – person group that will help you.

Try to confide in a close friend or a family member. You might feel ashamed, and may not want to open up at first, but the support that comes in return can be rewarding. Those women that shared their trouble trying to conceive said their friends and family were very supportive and 70% of them share their problems to people made the process easier.

Talk Things Out With Your Partner

Infertility can put a strain on your relationship. The GFK Roper survey that was carried out found that couples finding it difficult to get pregnant experiences a great deal of emotional upheaval. Couples should sit and talk things out. Have it in mind that each one of you is coping the best way you know you can.

Try to Empower Yourself

Infertility makes you feel like you no longer have control over your body, and your life. It is advisable to focus on what you can control. Learn the life style habits you know you can work on to boost your chance of conception – avoid smoking, limit caffeine and alcohol, go on with moderate exercise, and lose or gain weight so that your BMI is in the normal range.

Since infertility is an issue couple face, try and empower yourself and encourage your partner to do same.

DONT'S

Couples should not Lose Hope

Infertility is not a permanent crisis. Most couples who experience infertility do end up with their healthy baby. Research has shown that it doesn't have a permanent impact on the quality of your life.

Don't be Ashamed

Don't forget, this condition is a medical condition and is not permanent, and 8 million people in the country are going through this condition. Most couples with this condition feel ashamed, but you should not feel ashamed having fertility issues. 8 in 10 women said infertility makes them feel imperfect, and of the number of men said it makes them feel inadequate. The earlier you accept the cards you have been dealt, the faster you can get help and likely have your healthy, happy baby.

Don't Assume IVF is the Only Way out

 Most couples believe that if they don't luckily conceive on their own, IVF is the only option left for them to get pregnant.

The average price of an IVF is $12,400, the prospect can be intimidating. There is other less expensive and invasive ways to accomplish a healthy pregnancy, such as taking ovulation pills that are prescribe by your doctor.

Stop Blaming Yourself

Infertility is more common than you think. It is likely to be as a result from the male or female partner, and in some cases it's as a result from both. So don't waste your energy beating yourself up over what is out of your con troll. There is very little that couples can do about the cause of infertility as revealed by some medical experts.

CHAPTER SIX

Common Fertility Mistakes to Note When Trying to Get Pregnant

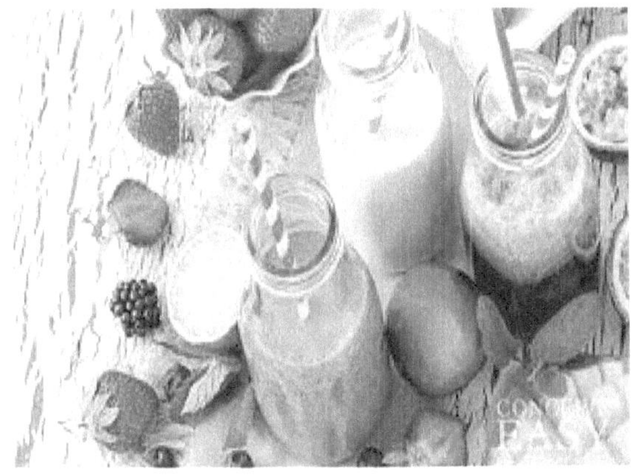

Couples should avoid these common mistakes when trying to conceive.

Are you guilty of some of these mistakes? Find out if you're and learn some cool fixes that could help you back to conceive.

Not knowing Your Actual Date of Ovulation

Most women have 28 days cycle, which means these women ovulation generally happens on day 14 of their cycle. Women have different cycles, so your cycle may be longer or shorter. To figure your exact ovulation date, you need to count 14 days back ward from the actual day you started your flow. You can make use of ovulation predictor tool to help you to know when you will ovulate next.

Waiting Too Long to get Pregnant

We know that you have a lot left in your mind to do (trying to establish a career, buying bigger house beefing up your saving etc.) Have it in mind that age waits for no one, and age is a factor in fertility. When you get to 35 years of age, then you have entered what is called "advanced maternal age," As you grow older, the risk of having trouble when trying to conceive and carrying a healthy pregnancy increases. According to Lobo, a woman's chances to conceive reduce by 50% between the ages of 20 – 40. If your relationship is stable and want a baby, don't wait just because you consider it not to be a problem to get pregnant later in life.

Just assume the Fertility Problem is From You

Most fertility investigation are carried out on women, but Lobo point out that 35% of the time, these problems can actually be attributed to the man. So if you find it difficult to conceive after a of trying to and are under the 35 years of age, you and your partner should see the doctor. Your doctor will carry out a semen analysis on your partner to

rule out any underlining issues on his
end.

Staying Too Long to See a Doctor

If you know your cycle is longer than
35 days or shorter than 25days, if you
are experiencing very painful or
heavy flows, or you have once had a
significant pelvic infection in the past,
it is better for you to see your
specialist to get everything checked
out. Make sure you put up to your
doctor's appointment, if you have
STDs history. If you feel you have
been exposed to one, it is better to
get checked to be sure.

Still Practicing Unhealthy Habits

Make sure you stay away from bad habits like drinking, smoking and drugs once you know you are pregnant. But have it in mind that lifestyle factors can still disturb your fertility too. To give up the above mentioned habits, make sure you consume a healthy diet, do exercise, get your weight into healthy range and ease up on caffeine.

Aiming on Sex Positions

Lifting your legs in the air or you bending into any other coital position of your choice to up your baby making chances, here are some news for you. The fact is, the man's sperm moves toward the woman's egg the moment he ejaculates. As remaining liquid that comes out after? It won't actually contain much sperm left in it. You can go ahead with your missionary – style or prop a pillow under your hips – but make sure you don't stress yourself too much.

Sex Every Single Day

Believe it or no, having sex every day can reduce your man's sperm count, which needs few days to rebound. Once you note your timing of ovulation, you continue to sex every other day, instead of having sex every single day during your fertile window.

Having Intercourse Only on the Day of Your Ovulation

When you are trying to get pregnant, timing matters a lot – but it doesn't mean you got only one chance shot at making a baby! An egg released during ovulation can survive in the fallopian tube for 12 – 24 hours. There, the egg meet with up with any sperm available, which can live in the woman's body for 3 days and sometimes up to 5 days, according to a specialist in New York City Jaime Knopman and co-founder of Truly-MD.com. It means your fertile window is potentially 6 days - the 4 days leading up to ovulation, the day in which you ovulate and the next day. And you are most fertile during the 2-3 days before your ovulation day and the main day of ovulation itself.

CHAPTER SEVEN
CONCLUSION

Nutrition helps to determine the successes of conceiving and also plays a vital role during pregnancy. Try and aim to achieve a healthy body weight, also maintain proper eating habit. Avoid harmful substances and lifestyle behaviors.

www.ingramcontent.com/pod-product-compliance
Lightning Source LLC
Chambersburg PA
CBHW031245130726
47988CB00008B/3239